Kidney Stones Guide

with Treatment and Prevention Tips

Contents

DISCLAIMER:

The information in this book is for informational purposes only. It is not intended to provide any sort of medical advice. If you require medical advice or medical treatment, consult your doctor. The author is not providing medical advice in any way and this information should not be taken as medical advice.

KIDNEY STONES: AN INTRODUCTION

The kidney is one of the key organs of human body that helps in the process of removing waste products away from the body by way of urine. Sometimes, the waste products are not dissolved and they remain in solid form in the kidney. Such crystals or lumps of waste products are referred to as Kidney stones. The size of the kidney stone varies from small, medium to large. The stones found in the kidney are either brown or yellow in color. Some stones may be smooth and brittle while some of them are hard.

Kidney stones sometimes may block the urinary track and thereby cause pain while passing urine. This has been one of the disorders present in human beings for centuries. As years pass by, the number of people suffering from this problem of kidney stones has shown a steady increase. This situation has been aggravated in the last decade due to wrong food habits.

The problem of kidney stones is common in adults rather than children. The most common type of kidney stone found in the human body contains calcium. Therefore, some changes in the intake of diet and fluid consumption will help dissolve these stone. Some types of kidney stones would dissolve without any treatment if you just focus on increasing your intake of water per day. However, complicated and stubborn stones must be removed through proper medication or surgery.

The human body is structured in such a way that the urinary system is highly dependent on the digestive system. The Kidneys process the waste materials passed on from the digestive system. Any minor problem in the digestive system like diarrhea or constipation could trigger off the formation of kidney stone.Hence, the medical experts always insist that we need to be aware of what we eat and we drink, as a small change in that may go a long way .

CAUSES FOR KIDNEY STONE

There are no definite reasons for the formation of Kidney stones. Sometimes certain food habits may cause stones. People who consume rich animal protein diet, low fibrous food combined with fewer intakes of fluids are at more risk of being a victim of Kidney stone. Eating too much of purine foods like fish, meat and poultry may sometimes cause kidney stones. In few cases kidney stone formation may just be due to more sugar consumption.

Men are more likely to get kidney stones than women. Family history may also be a cause for kidney stone. Some other reasons for developing kidney stones are as follows:

Gout

Gout is a condition, which cause an increase in the level of uric acid in blood and thereby deposits lumps of uric acid in the form of kidney stone. Gout may be developed by obesity, alcohol intake, high blood pressure and some malfunction in kidney.

HyperCalciuria

This is the main reason for kidney stones for most people. The term Hypercalciuria means that there is a presence of high calcium content in urine. In many cases, a large quantity of calcium is absorbed from the diet consumed and is excreted in the urine.

Inflammatory bowel diseases

People suffering from inflammatory bowel disease may have higher chances of getting kidney stones. This disease will initially affect the intestine and then the liver, eyes and other organs. In rare cases, it may cause kidney stones too.

Other diseases

Urinary tract infections, kidney disorders and other metabolic disorders may cause Kidney stones. Hyperparathyroidism can lead to stone formation. A popular hereditary disease known as the renal tubular acidosis could also assist in the formation of kidney stones.

Cystinuria and Hyperoxaluria are some of the disorders that may cause kidney stones. Cystinuria is a condition where lot of amino acid cystine is deposited which do not dissolve in the urine and thus lead to stone formation. Hyperoxaluria is a condition where the urine contains more oxalate than the level that can be dissolved. Oxalate is a salt that will be formed as crystals and thus cause kidney stones.

Sometimes intestinal bypass surgery may lead to kidney stone formation. People who are undergoing treatment for HIV infection with a medicine called protease inhibitor indinavir may be considered high risk.

People who are living in warm climates may also have the risk of getting kidney stones. Over dosage of Vitamin D or taking too much of vitamin supplements can cause stones, too.

SYMPTOMS OF KIDNEY STONES

Most the kidney stones do present themselves with any symptoms. However, if the size of the stone is large, then it could lead to blockage in the urinary tract resulting in severe pain while passing urine. In such condition, the person may feel pain in the lower abdomen. He may feel nausea accompanied with vomiting.

Sometimes Blood may be seen in the urine. This is because the stone will irritate the ureter and cause blood. However all the cases with blood in urine do not really indicate the presence of Kidney stones. Some other reasons may also cause blood spots in urine.

Frequent and painful urination may also be a symptom of the presence of kidney stone. Many people feel stinging or burning sensations while passing urine. Tenderness in kidney, abdomen and Urinary tract infection may also be signs of kidney stones.

If there is a foul smell along with pus in urine, then there is a strong indication that there is a stone present in the kidney. If all these symptoms and chills persist along with any of the above symptoms then the person should seek medical help immediately.

HOW TO DIAGNOSE KIDNEY STONES?

You can come to know the presence of kidney stone through self diagnosis. This should immediately be done when you feel extreme pain while passing urine. However, the doctor will confirm the same through certain tests. Such tests include the following:

Spiral Computed topography

Spiral Computed topography, also popularly known as CT scan is the best test to diagnose the presence of a kidney stone. By using this technology, one can get a thorough scan of the ureter and kidneys.

The results obtained through this test are accurate. It takes more time to take this test in comparison with other tests. Intravenous Pyelogram (IVP) will help to view the position of urinary tract.

This X-ray test is taken after giving an injection of certain dye into the vein in the arm. A series of X-ray tests is taken at regular intervals to diagnose the kidney stones.

An injection is required to pass certain dye into the vein. This will help in getting clear view of the stones.

In addition to the IVP or CT scan, one can also opt for Retrograde Pyelogram tests. In this test, there is no particular injection given in the vein. Instead, the dye is injected through the tubes that help in carrying urine from the kidney.

Another test to diagnose kidney stones is by the method of Urinalysis. Through this test one could determine the complete details of the components in the urine. This will help to test the pH level in urine. For example if the pH level is four, then the urine is strongly acidic, 7 is neutral and 9 is strongly alkaline. Apart from this urine test, it will also help to test if blood is present in urine.

An abdominal x-ray will help in providing the clear picture of kidney, urinary bladder and the tube connecting the kidney and bladder. This will therefore identify kidney stones.

Ultra sound tests use high frequency sound waves to give diagnostically oriented pictures of internal organs. They can detect stones in the ureter. However, it is not possible to diagnose small stones with the help of this test. This test is mainly used to detect kidney stones in a pregnant woman.

Who can diagnose kidney stones?

If you feel any kind of symptoms of kidney stone then you should immediately seek the help of your family doctor. He can diagnose whether you have a kidney stone and if so what is the type of kidney stone and so on. An urologist can also help you in kidney stone diagnosis. He can also provide treatment of diseases in urinary tract for both men and women.

Once you had passed kidney stones with the treatment by a specialist, then you need to get another test to diagnose whether there are any possibilities of getting the stones back and how to avoid this if so.

TREATMENTS FOR KIDNEY STONES

Most kidney stones can be cured by taking medication.

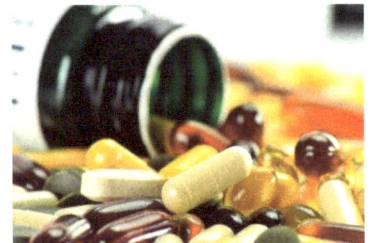

If the stone is small, then it may just pass out in urine. Taking adequate fluid and pain control pills will be sufficient for removing such stones. Normally 5 out of 10 small stones will pass automatically without taking any medication.

While the treatment is on, consumption of grape juice may increase the complications of kidney stone. Therefore, you should not take this while receiving treatment. Instead you could take extra two glasses of water daily to remove the small kidney stones.

The doctor will prescribe some medicines to get relief from stones. Calcium channel blockers will help in removing small stones. However, it may have some side effects. If you have severe pain then your doctor will prescribe non-steroidal anti-inflammatory to relieve pain. Sometimes pain control medicines will cause side effects like vomiting, drowsiness, constipation etc. So it is better to take such medication after consulting your doctor.

If the pain is more and uncontrollable even after taking pain control pills then medical treatment becomes a necessity. Your doctor will decide which treatment will be more suitable for you after analyzing your age, family history and so on. Some common medical treatments are as follows:

Extracorporeal Shock wave Lithotripsy

This treatment uses shock waves that will enter your body easily and will help break the kidney stones into smaller pieces so that they can be thrown out of the body through the urinary tract easily. This treatment never causes any injury to your body. However, the doctor will give you some sedatives like anesthesia which can be local or general.

If the stone is somewhat large then the doctor will use a tube with a mesh called stent to keep the ureter open. This will help in passing the stones without blocking the ureter. This treatment requires just an hour and you can return home on the same day.

This treatment is suitable when the stone size is anywhere between 4 mm to 2.5 cm. Although it does not cause any pain, pregnant women, persons suffering from kidney infections, bleeding disorders etc are not advised to go for this treatment. It is not safe for those with pacemakers as well.

Percutaneous nephrolithotomy:

This method involves the treatment of inserting a small telescope into the kidney through a cut in the patient's back. Then the surgeon will remove the small stones. If the stone is large, then he will break it down into pieces and then remove it. This method is used when the stone is large and could not be removed by extracorporeal shock wave treatment.

Ureteroscopy

In this method, the surgeon will insert a thin telescope called ureteroscope into the urethra. But he will not make any incision in the body for inserting the telescope. This will help him to identify the location of the kidney stone. Then he will use small forceps to remove the kidney stones. It is easy to remove smaller stones. However, for larger stones, the surgeon will have to break down to pieces first.

Breaking down the larger stones is a difficult process. There are several instruments available to break the stone into small pieces. In fact, most of the surgeons prefer laser in this process. But Uteroscopy is not possible if the person had already had surgery in abdomen or pelvis. Any injury in ureter may also prevent the surgeon to give this treatment.

Ureteroscopy is the best method for removing kidney stones. It proves to be successful for more than 95% of people. The treatment does not require long hours. The patient can return home the next day itself.

HOW TO PREVENT KIDNEY STONES?

Every year millions of people are affected by the kidney stone disorder. Some changes in life style and food habits may help in preventing the disease. You should avoid taking excessive acidic foods. Avoiding unhealthy diets that include large quantities of white flour, tea, coffee, cocoa etc will prevent kidney stones.

In most of the cases, kidney stones are formed by high calcium and high oxalate level. This can be controlled by taking balanced diet. Taking a lot of milk based food products, alkaline foods and vitamin supplements may cause kidney stones as well. Extreme intake of vitamin c or its supplements will cause stones. You can avoid such foods or take in small quantities.

Drinking adequate water will help in preventing kidney stones. However, taking in more salt and processed food will cause stone formation in kidneys; hence this should be carefully avoided. High fiber diets are also very helpful in the prevention of kidney stones.

Limiting the usage of rich oxalate food will also help you in staying away from kidney stone.

Healthy and balanced diet will help in preventing kidney stones. Fruits and vegetables are rich in fiber which should be included in your daily diet. Sometimes metabolic disorder may also cause kidney stone. Hence add more fluid in your regular diet.

People who receive treatment for removing kidney stones will have 40 % chance for getting stones again. However, eating right food and taking lot of fluid will help in preventing reappearance of kidney stones.

Normally men are more likely to suffer from kidney stone rather than women. 80% of them have excess calcium oxalate in the urine. Preventing dehydration and diarrhea may help preventing kidney stones. Ginger ale, lemon juice and fresh fruit juices can prevent stone formation.

Caffeine products may increase the risk of kidney stones. Hence avoiding coffee, tea, cola etc may help in preventing the disorder to a large extent. Restricting acidic foods will also help you in avoiding kidney stones. And you should not take vitamin supplements excessively without the prescription of your doctor. Excessive vitamins will only harm your health instead of boosting it.

If you have any doubt that you may have a kidney stone, then you should reduce the intake of dairy products. Taking calcium in pill form will increase the risk of stone formation. Taking reduced meat, fish and poultry will also help you to reduce the risk. Even though the kidney stone disorder is treatable, Prevention is the better than cure.

If you want to prevent kidney stones and decrease the risk of having any kidney stones, then you can opt for a 24-hour urine test. This test will identify the small stones in the initial stage itself. Then your doctors will probably advise you to take some drugs like potassium citrate, magnesium citrate, allopurinol and so on depending upon the type of stone. Early medication is always better since it will help the sufferer avoid any surgical treatment.

KIDNEY STONES IN ADULTS

Normally adults aged over 20 years are more likely to be affected by kidney stones. This may affect men above 40s more. Women are likely to be affected when they reach 50 years of age particularly during the time of menopause. It is a painful disease. However it is not a new disorder. In fact, it is proven that kidney stone were prevalent 7000 years before now.

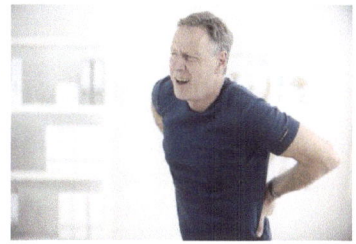

A recent study shows that 10 % of people experience the pain due to kidney stones in their life time. Some may have small stones that will be dissolved without any medication. But large stones need medication including surgical treatment.

In fact, kidney stones are developed from crystals that separate from the urine. Normally the content in the urine consists of chemicals which prevent crystals. However such chemicals may fail to work properly for some people.

There are so many reasons for this stone formation. Hereditary conditions may also cause kidney stones, for instance. And whites are generally more affected with this disease than blacks.

Recent research shows that some people have more chances of getting kidney stones than others.

The list as such follows:

- A person with a family history of kidney stones may have the risk of developing stones.
- About 70% of people around the globe are affected with kidney stones when they have a hereditary disease called renal tubular acidosis.
- Persons suffering from frequent urinary tract infections may also have the risk of stone formation.
- Persons experiencing chronic inflammatory in the bowels may also have the possibility of developing stones.
- A disorder of uric acid metabolism, gout and blockage in urinary tract may cause kidney stones.
- Calcium antacids intake will increase the chance of getting kidney stones in adults.
- People who had passed kidney stones may have the risk of getting stones again.
- Cystic kidney diseases and hyperparathyroidism in adults may cause stone formation.
- Struvite stones may affect people with urinary tract infection. But such cases are rare.
- People who are taking treatment for HIV infection with protease inhibitor indinavir also have the risk of promoting kidney stones.
- People who are suffering from cancer or a disease called sarcoidosis have the risk of getting calcium stones in kidney.
- Persons having one kidney or abnormal shape kidney also are at risk.

FOODS THAT MAY CAUSE KIDNEY STONES:

In many cases wrong food habits are one of the main reasons that trigger the formation of kidney stone. Many people are under the impression that the excessive intake of soft drinks will result in obesity and indigestion alone. But it is a prime factor for the formation of kidney stones. The acidity and mineral imbalances in soft drinks will increase the risk of kidney stone development.

Eating lot of meat will cause uric acid stones in kidneys. Excessive sugar intake will cause not only diabetes but also kidney stones. Sometimes high protein diet may also result in stone formation. Red meat, fish and poultry should be taken in lesser quantity and in less frequency. Coffee, soda, cocoa, tea should be avoided or take one or two times daily. White flour should be avoided to control stone formation.

Though scientists have specified that there is no direct connection between food and kidney stones, you should avoid any food that may cause allergies. Food allergies tend to cause ingestion and that in turn may cause inflammatory bowel disorders. This again will cause kidney stones.

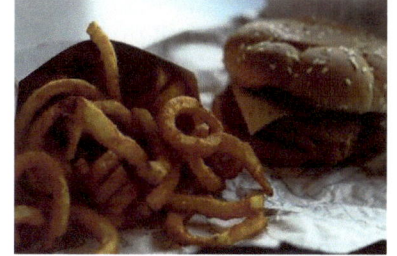

Uric acid may cause kidney stones. It is present in food like sweet bread, liver and kidney. Therefore such foods should be avoided. Spinach may also be avoided as it increases the risk of promoting kidney stones.

A dairy diet can be replaced with vegetable protein diet like beans and soy to be more beneficial. Of course, check with your family doctor first before any dieting is done.

You can avoid the above foods and diets that may increase the risk of kidney stone development. Again, check with your family doctor first about the right diet for you and your family.

Drinking plenty of water can help prevent kidney stones. In fact, small stones will be dissolved if you take in more water regularly.

Lemonade is proven to be a good remedy for dissolving kidney stones. Generally kidney stones are formed when the urine lacks enough substance to prevent them. Such substance mainly includes citrate. Normally doctors will prescribe potassium citrate in pill form to remove small stones in kidney. Instead of taking pills, taking adequate lemonade will help you in passing kidney stones in a natural way. Always remember natural ways do not have any side effects.

You can include calcium in your diet. Initially you could consume vegetables and fruits which have a natural calcium content in them instead of taking calcium supplements. Green peas, pumpkin, tomatoes, cauliflower, cabbage etc can be included. Fresh fruits like guava, water melon, papaya, pine apple etc can also be taken.

TYPES OF KIDNEY STONES

Kidney stones are classified according to their composition. Such classification is essential to start the treatment. There are 5 types of kidney stones. They are as follows...

Calcium stones

This is the major type of stone found in 50% of the people who suffer from kidney stone disorder. Kidney stones normally found in persons who are taking excessive calcium particularly in pill form. People who are suffering from recurrent stone formation in kidney are more likely affected calcium oxalate stones.

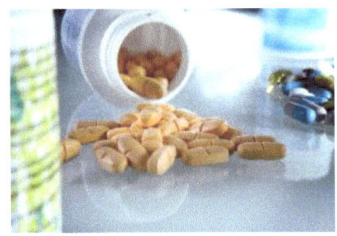 Calcium and vitamins in pill form tend to aggravate kidney stone formation. We all know that vitamin D is essential in absorbing calcium. This is good for bones. But excessive absorption of vitamin D will only harm your health by producing Calcium stones.

If you are diagnosed with these types of stones, then you should limit the consumption of dairy products, meat and poultry. Instead start taking low calcium high fiber diet.

Allopurinal is proven to be the most effective drug for calcium stone sufferers. However if the drug shows any side effects in any of the patients, then he/ she should stop consuming the medications.

Uric Acid Stones

Uric acid stones are another common type found in kidney stone sufferers. This will occur when the urine has a high concentration of uric acid or the uric acid is present in such a form which is easily dissolvable in water.

People having high risk of uric acid stones

- People who receive Chemotherapy treatment for curing cancer have more concentration of uric acid in urine than normal people.
- People who live in hot and arid areas and one who do not consume at least eight to ten glasses of water may have the chance of frequent dehydration. They will lead to low volume of urine output and thereby increase the risk of uric acid stones.
- People who have inflammatory bowel disorders or those who have the problem of chronic diarrhea have the problem of low pH urine and low volume of urine. This in turn will increase the stone formation.

Symptoms of Uric acid stones

The person suffering from uric acid stones will experience extreme pain and will also notice blood in urine like any other types of kidney stones. Hence a complete diagnosis will only help in recognizing the type of kidney stone. Normally uric acid stones will not be seen in X-ray. A CT scan and 24 hours urine test is necessary to identify the stone.

Treatment for uric acid stones

Uric acid stones though cause severe pain are not difficult to remove. Drinking adequate fluid along with increase in urine pH level is sufficient to pass uric acid stones. Normally shock wave treatments are not required for removing this type of stone.

How to prevent uric acid stones

Taking more than 2 liters of water daily will help in preventing uric acid stones. Fresh fruits will help in raising the urine pH level by supplying potassium bicarbonate or potassium citrate to the body.

If you do not get effective results in removing stones by the above simplest approach, then your doctor will advise you to take allopurinol drugs.

Struvite stones

Struvite stones are also described as infection stones since they occur mainly due to urinary tract infections. These stones will grow fast and will occupy large parts of the kidney. Even though lots of antibiotics are available nowadays, this infection stone is prevalent in some 15 to 20 % of kidney stone sufferers.

The bacteria that are producing urinary tract infections and thereby struvite stones are proteus and klebsiella. Any conditions that cause urinary tract infection with bacteria have the ability to produce ammonia which will be a key factor in struvite stone formation. Since bladder may have some urine stagnant, the possibility of bacteria growing is more.

Symptoms of struvite stone

Struvite stone does not really show any symptoms like other stones. Mild pain and blood in urine may be seen. However these symptoms can be normally associated with urinary tract infection only. Recurrent infection may be a symptom of struvite stone.

How to diagnose the Struvite stones?

If you have recurrent urinary tract infection then you should go for x-ray or CTscan. This will clearly help in identifying the type of stone. Urine test that shows high pH level more than 7 will also state the formation of struvite stone. A microscopic test that shows crystals in urine will also indicate Struvite stones.

What are the risks involved with this stone?

As already told, this stone will grows at a very fast pace and can cause infections frequently. Sometimes it may also cause acute kidney failure. Normally frequent infection will cause chronic kidney failure.

What are the treatments available to treat Struvite stones?

The complication of this stone makes it indispensable to take treatment as early as possible. Medication will not be successful for more people in removing this stone. Extra corporeal shock wave lithotripsy (ESWL) is useful in removing small stones. If the stone is difficult to remove by ESWL method then percutaneous nephrolithotomy can be used.

In some rare cases ESWL is used after percutaneous nephrolithotomy to remove smaller pieces of stones. For larger stones, open surgery is required.

After removing the stones, follow up is required at regular intervals to confirm new stones have not been formed.

How to prevent Struvite stones?

Struvite stone formation can be prevented by restricting or treating urinary tract infection. Once you have struvite stones, then you should completely remove the stones in any of the above methods. This is important because struvite stones will also cause calcium stone formation and then in turn may lead to kidney failure.

Cystine stones

Cystine stones are not common since their formation highly relates to a rare disease called Cystinuria. This problem occurs mainly in children and young adults. Children having family history of this stone are more likely to be affected by this disease.

Causes for Cystine stone formation

It is a normal fact that amino acids are filtered in the urine. However, a normal kidney can reabsorb them from urine and transfer them in the blood. In cystinuria, the kidneys fail to reabsorb from the urine the cystine amino acids. Therefore, cystine will be dissolved in the urine so as to form crystals. This in turn will result in the growth of stones.

How to diagnose this stone?

Unlike other stones, the Cystine stone will induce continuous pain. Children affected by this disease will complain about severe pain. This is a clear symptom of this stone. X-ray will identify the stone but not that much clear as calcium stone. However, IVP or CT scan will clearly diagnose the stone.

An x-ray is enough to diagnose small stones.

Treatment for Cystine stones

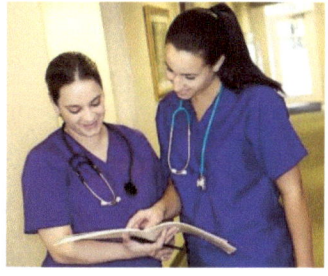
Treatment for cystine stones is essential like other stones since it may cause not only pain but also urine infections and sometimes kidney failure. Traditional treatment involves taking adequate fluids. Taking 3 liters extra water will help in dissolving the cystine stones. Sodium intake must be reduced. Usually cystine stone is the result of high pH level in urine. The pH level must be reduced to pass the stone.

Taking plenty of water will be more beneficial. Of course it is the cheapest form of medicine.

Medication

Sometimes the above traditional methods may not be effective. Therefore people may require medication to remove the stone or stones. Drugs available for this disorder are penicillamine, tiopronin and captopril. Pencillamine is available everywhere but it may cause few side effects. Tiopronin is the best drug available all over the world and it is proven to be effective in removing the stones. Captopril will cause fewer side effects than the other two but it is not that much effective.

If the above medication does not provide any positive results then the doctor can suggest some other procedures. But in fact the shock waves do not provide successful results particularly if the stone is large. The large stones are first broken down into smaller pieces and then pencilamine is injected directly into the kidney. This will help in dissolving the small pieces of stones.

Cystine stone is one of the most complicated problems and so traditional treatment should be continued up to 1 or 2 years and the medication must be continued for six months after treatment. This is important because the possibility of getting stones again is higher here. People suffering from multiple stones are at higher risk as it may lead to kidney failure and then there is no other option left other than undergoing a kidney transplant which is the last possible way to cure the disease.

Drug stone

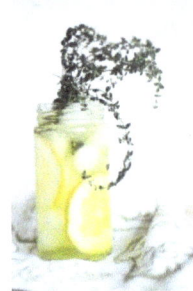 People who are under medication for any ailment are also under risk of kidney stones as the drugs taken to cure that disease may form crystals and then such crystals can grow as stones.

People taking treatment for HIV infection with the drug called protease inhibitor indinavir and triamterene are also considered at having a risk of drug stone formation.

Although we have divided the kidney stones into 5 types, some kidney stones will be formed by combining one or two types. One type of stone formation will tend to form another type also.

Shapes of kidney stones

The size and shape of the kidney stone normally varies from person to person. However it will not look like a smooth, round ball. The shape will be irregular. The size may vary from millimeters to few centimeters. The color, texture etc will also vary from person to person.

The most common colors of kidney stones are yellow and brown. But gold, tan and black may also be the colors of the kidney stones. The normal shape of a kidney stone may be round, jagged or branch like. The texture may also differ according to the composition of the stone.

HOW TO REMOVE KIDNEY STONES?

Kidney stones though painful are not difficult to remove. You need not fear that all stones require surgical treatment. Sometimes small stones will be dissolved in the urine without any medication. But, when the stone obstructs the urinary tract and cause pain, then it is necessary to remove the stones through surgery.

Natural treatment for removing kidney stones:

Uri flow is a non-prescription medicine which actively removes kidney stones. It directly hits the chemical composition and thus dissolves the stones to pass. It will not create any pain in the removal process. In fact it helps in cleaning the urinary tract. It helps in preventing inflammation and urine infection. It effectively prevents the reoccurrence of stones.

If you leave kidney stones untreated then these may damage the kidneys. Uri flow is mainly aiming at breaking down the stone into pieces and thereby flushes out the pieces in the urine. It will not cause any irritation. There is no risk in this medicine. It is 100 % guaranteed by a number of doctors.

Other drugs used in removing kidney stones are as follows:

Calcium and uric acid stones can be controlled by giving the drug named allopurinol. Hyperuricosiria can be effectively controlled by this medicine.

Hypercalciuria will lead to calcium stone formation. Therefore doctors will prescribe drugs to control hypercalciuria. The drug containing hydrochlorothiazide will help in decreasing the calcium amount released by the kidney.

The cystine stones can be controlled by taking adequate fluid. However doctors may advice to take drugs in addition to fluid intake. Such drugs like Thiola and cuprimine will be helpful in preventing cystine in urine.

As briefly mentioned earlier above struvite stones are caused by urinary tract infections, doctors will prescribe drugs containing acetohydroxamic acid. This will act as an anti biotic and thus prevents stone growth.

The above mentioned drugs are easily available every where and so you need not fear that kidney stones will stop your normal life. The disease though slightly painful can be curable with drugs in most of the cases.

SOME HOME REMEDIES TO TREAT KIDNEY STONES

Apart from the medication, you can also take some home remedies to dissolve kidney stones. Ayurvedic herbs will also help in dissolving kidney stones quickly without any pain.

Some home remedies for removing kidney stones are as follows:

- Take two figs and boil it in one cup of water for few seconds. Take this regularly in the morning in the empty stomach. A glass full of grape fruit juice without sugar or a cup of lemonade daily will also help in dissolving kidney stones.

- Have a glass of lemon juice daily to avoid the formation of stones in Kidney.

- Approximately 90% of people who experience the presence of stones in their kidney do so due to excessive calcium intake. Thus reducing dairy products and avoiding calcium supplements will be more beneficial in removing stones.

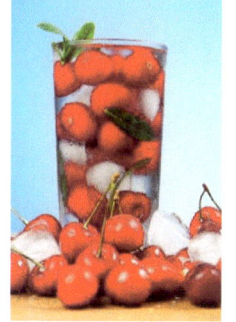

- High oxalate foods may cause calcium oxalate stones. Tea, coffee, chocolates, spinach etc have high oxalate. You can restrict the usage of such products to get rid of stone problems.

- Though very tempting, there is a strong need to avoid coffee as this aggravates the situation of kidney stone formation.

- Drink a glass of tart cherry juice. When drinking cherry juice look for 100% pure tart cherry juice concentrate. You can find 100% cherry juice concentrate from Traverse Bay Farms located in Northern Michigan.

- Watermelon and pomegranates can be taken either as fruits or as juices to pass kidney stones. These fruits will also reduce the acidity in urine.

- Pomegranate Juice is quite effective in preventing kidney stone formation.

- Basil juice and honey can help in dissolving the granules in kidney. Pomegranate seeds have the power of dissolving kidney stones. Take the seeds, dry and powder it. Take one tea spoon of such powder daily adding it to horse gram soup.

- Basil juice helps in relieving kidney stone symptoms.

- French beans will also help in removing kidney stones.

- Make a juice of radish leaves and take two teaspoon of the same regularly. This may help to a great extent in dissolving kidney stones.

- Cranberry juice and ripe apples have the power to remove kidney stones.

- Tomato juice with pepper and a pinch of salt in the empty stomach will remove kidney stones.

- Onion with a little sugar will have its own effect of reducing kidney stone problem. The most important benefit of these home remedies is that they never cause any side effects.

- Healthy and balanced diets along with adequate fluid intake can surely help in dissolving kidney stones. And avoid smoking when you have any doubt of getting kidney stone formation.

SURGICAL TREATMENT TO REMOVE KIDNEY STONES

Most of the kidney stones that people have are small and can be dissolved with some natural remedies or through medication. However, some large stones are difficult to remove with medication. Such complicated stones require surgical treatment.

Surgical treatment is also required to break down the large stones into pieces. Such small pieces will be later on removed by taking drugs.

What are the types of surgical treatment available for removing kidney stones?

Ureteroscopy

In this method, a small telescope is inserted into the urethra and passed through the bladder to reach the stone. Once the stone is located then the surgeon will remove the stone with the small basket attached with the telescope. If it is not possible to remove the stone, then he will break it down into pieces. Ureteroscopy is done after giving local anesthesia to the patient.

Lithotripsy

If the stone is located in the kidney or upper urethra, then Lithotripsy can be used to remove the stone. This method involves a small instrument which will break down the stone into number of small pieces. The small pieces will then be passed on in the urine. Though this method is effective, it is not suitable for those persons who are suffering from large stones or those who have any other medical problems.

Ultrasonic lithotripsy

This method resembles the lithotripsy method but with a small difference. This method uses sound waves to break down the stone. The sound waves are inserted into the urethra through an electronic probe. The surgeon will then remove the small pieces of stones or they will get removed while the patient passes urine.

Electro hydraulic lithotripsy

In this method the shock waves are generated with the help of electricity and that will be inserted into urethra through a flexible probe. This method is highly efficient in breaking down kidney stones anywhere in the urinary system. General anesthesia is required for the patient to do this surgery.

Extra corporeal shock wave lithotripsy

This method uses highly impulsive shock waves to break down stones anywhere in the urinary system. In this method the surgeon will break down the stone into small sand like granules which will then be passed on by the patient in the urine. The surgery requires one hour. Local or general anesthesia will be given to the patient for doing this surgery. This method should not be used for removing large stones or stuvite stones. This method is strictly prohibited for treating a pregnant woman.

Percutaneous Nephrostolithotomy

This method is performed by the surgeon after giving local anesthesia or intravenous sedation. A needle and guide wire is used to identify the exact location of the stone. Once the stone location is identified, the surgeon will use some surgical instruments like forceps to remove the stone. This method is highly effective in removing large and medium stones than any other method. However, the patient will have required hospitalization for two weeks. Then he/she can start his\ her regular activity.

Open surgery

A doctor will suggest open surgery for the patient in some rare cases. Such conditions require open surgery since other methods do not provide successful results. Here a cut is made in the patient's back and the stone is removed through the cut. The patient will be given general anesthesia. He will require lot days in hospitalization in this method. Then he can return to normal life. But nowadays open surgery for kidney stones is rarely a practice.

Risk of open surgery to remove kidney stones

There are some risks in open surgery for removing kidney stones. Such risks include severe bleeding, risk of anesthesia and infection. Due to theses risks and the introduction of percutaneous nephrostolithotomy, extra corporeal shock wave lithotripsy etc eliminates the need for open surgery in kidney.

Though there are some inconveniences in surgical treatments, they completely eliminate the stones present in any part of the urinary system. Therefore kidney stones though painful, can be curable with any of the above method. Your doctor will decide upon one of the methods that is suitable for you.

He will decide after considering your medical condition, age, family history and about the nature of the stone. Most of the surgical treatment requires hospitalization from one hour to two weeks. Then you can resume to your normal life. However doctor may advice you to continue some medication for few days.

KIDNEY STONES IN WOMEN

Normally men are more likely to be affected by kidney stones than women. The reason is yet unknown. Only 20 % of the total kidney stone sufferers are women. However women suffering from kidney stones may face pain and discomfort.

Women who take rich oxalate foods, take inadequate water and fluid are likely to suffer from kidney stone formation. Every year the number of American women suffering from kidney stones is increasing. Wrong food habits and care free lifestyles are the main reasons for this.

Symptoms of Kidney Stones in Women

The main symptom of kidney stones in women is the acute pain. The pain will be more when the stone blocks the urethra. Most of the women complaint that the pain is similar to the labor pain they had experienced while giving birth. However when the stone stops migrating then it may not produce pain. But it will cause severe infection, damage kidney functions or stop kidney functions.

Another important symptom is that women may feel pain at the time of menstruation in the lower abdomen. However they may not identify the pain with kidney stones.

If the pain is followed by fever, dullness, vomiting, nausea etc then they should immediately seek medical help. This is important because these symptoms are closely associated with kidney stones and early diagnosis can help to reduce the severity of the disease.

What are the causes for kidney stones in women?

Low intake of fruits and vegetable is the main reason for kidney stone formation in women. High protein diet and calcium supplements in pill form may increase the chance of stone formation.

Urinary tract infection is the main reason for forming stuvite stones. Such infection is common in women than men. Though men are more likely to be affected by kidney stones four times more than women, a recent study show that the risk of women getting kidney stone formation is increasing.

Every year the number of American women affected by kidney stones is increasing due to wrong food habits and sedentary lifestyles. Women above 40 years of age and women who are approaching their menopause years have more chances of getting kidney stones than other young women.

How to prevent Kidney stones in women?

As the risk of kidney stone formation is increasing in women nowadays, they should learn to take some preventive measures.

Such prevention methods include the following:

- Drink more water and sugar-free fluids daily.
- Add more fresh fruits, including and vegetables that are rich in vitamins and minerals to your diet. These are also rich in fiber which will help in metabolic activities. Note that metabolic disorders may also cause kidney stones.
- Eat dried fruit including dried tart cherries, pomegranate seeds and blueberries.
- If you have any infection, fever, chills, extreme pain in back or lower abdomen, then you should seek medical help immediately. You can take some pain control medicine after consulting your doctor.
- Women are more likely to get calcium stones. Oxalate rich foods can increase the level of calcium. Hence women should limit high oxalate foods like coffee, chocolates, spinach, tea etc.
- Taking calcium supplements must be avoided. Vitamin D is good for health and it enhances the calcium absorption. But excessive vitamin D will lead to calcium stone formation.
- Drinking tea often can prompt stone formation. Instead of drinking tea, you can instead make lemon tea which will help in reducing such risks.

Next to calcium stone, stuvite stones also affect women. This is because women experience more problems of urinary tract infections more than men do. Therefore, women should take preventative steps to avoid and treat such infections promptly, for example, by wiping from the front to back will be beneficial rather than cleaning from back to front. This will surely help in preventing urinary tract infections and thereby stop stuvite stone growth.

You should not hesitate to seek medical help if you have pain or infection. Urine tests and a health exam can help you in diagnosing stones, if there are any. And early diagnosis can help the doctor and you in curing the diseases fast.

Your doctor can prescribe some medication to prevent calcium stones and uric acid stone formation.

WHAT ARE THE RISKS INVOLVED FOR WOMEN SUFFERING FROM KIDNEY STONES?

The risks associated with the kidney stones for women are almost same like those for men. Obesity may increase the risk of kidney stone formation for women; kidney stones affect women more during their pregnancy. This is because women tend to take more calcium during pregnancy but their kidneys do not have the capacity to handle the excessive calcium. Therefore they have the risk of getting Calcium stones. However such cases are rare. About one in 1500 pregnant women has the chance of getting kidney stones.

Obesity and weight gain may cause kidney stones. Women who are obese have the greater risk of getting kidney stones. 90% of women who are obese are at risk of kidney stone than the normal woman. Beverage intake will increase the risk of kidney stone formation in women. Women who had removed their ovaries also have the risk of getting kidney stone.

Risks involved for women with kidney stones are as follows.

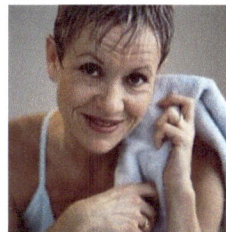

Pregnant women are likely to be affected by kidney stones. Giving treatment at this stage would be slightly critical as it might affect the womb inside. The risk is the same if you leave it untreated. Pregnant women who have kidney stones have the risk of preterm delivery over pregnant women with no kidney stone history. Any small stones can be removed with the help of medication. However large stones require surgical treatment that is strictly prohibited for pregnant women. Hence the risk of pregnant women with kidney stones is always more.

Though the risk of kidney stone in younger women is less than older women, wrong food habits will promote kidney stone formation.

HOW TO CONTROL THE RISK OF KIDNEY STONE IN WOMEN?

It is very important for women to stay fit and healthy in order to avoid the occurrence of kidney stones. Obesity is one of the major causes that can increase the risk of kidney stone formation in women. Women don't necessarily need to be very slender or very athletic for this purpose. Women have to maintain a balanced nutritional plan along with a regular exercise regime to control the risk of kidney stone occurrence.

Most people don't drink adequate amounts of fluids every day. A person has to drink nearly 8 to 10 glasses of pure drinking water to help maintain a proper PH level in the body. Drinking fluids helps maintain blood pressure as well as body temperature. It will also help you flush out all the toxins out of your body thus, reducing the chances of kidney stone formation.

Women tend to take plenty of over-the-counter calcium supplements as they begin to age. It is definitely not advisable to consume calcium, vitamin D or vitamin C supplements without consulting your physician first, as excess consumption of such vitamins can lead to formation of kidney stones. Pain pills as well as antipyretics should also be taken under proper medical guidance.

Some researches have indicated that intake of vitamin B6 in excess quantities by women, tends to cause kidney stones. Women require only 2 mg of vitamin B6 every day and this quantity must not exceed unless prescribed by a physician. Diet rich in sodium and high oxalate content foods such as chocolates, tea, green leafy vegetables will raise the risk of kidney stone formation in women as well as men. Such type of foodstuff should be taken in appropriate quantities to maintain the oxalate levels in the body.

Be careful about your medication and never consume expired or tainted pills.

As women age, they have to increase their daily calcium intake, but as excess calcium may cause kidney stone formation, precautions have to be taken regarding the dosages of calcium supplements.

Some causes of kidney stones occurrence in women that cannot be controlled:

- Postmenopausal women with low estrogen levels have a higher risk of developing kidney stones.
- Women, who have had to remove their ovaries, are also prone to kidney stone formations. Kidney stones can also occur if this condition is inherited from previous generations.
- Women with high diabetes, inflammatory bowel diseases along with prolonged urinary tract infections have higher chances of getting kidney stones.
- Sometimes abnormal pH level in urine cannot be controlled by diet or medication and is bound to cause kidney stones in a long run if not checked at initial stages.

IS THERE ANY POSSIBILITY OF REOCCURENCE OF KIDNEY STONES AFTER TREATMENT?

If the kidney stones are surgically removed, then the patient is made to stay at the hospital or the medical facility for nearly 2 weeks to undergo various tests and post-surgical treatments. During this time, the patient is frequently tested to detect any fragments of the kidney stones that may be left unchecked in any part of the urinary system.

Many people who have received treatment via surgery or any other method may face reoccurrence of kidney stones. To prevent kidney stones formation, certain alterations in diet, lifestyle and medication have to be done.

There are some people, who are widely susceptible for frequent reoccurrence of kidney stones. Clinical researches claim that a person, who has been suffering from kidney stones, faces a fifty percent chance of getting them again. Whereas, post-treatment, there is always a 15% chance of kidney stone reoccurrence.

To lower the chances of reoccurrence of kidney stones after surgical or medical treatments certain precautionary measures have to be followed. If kidney stones are a frequent occurrence in your family, there is chance that even you might experience them in a long run.

The precautions stated below should be taken care of even by those individuals who have never had kidney stones in their live, but have family members with a history of kidney stones.

- Have your physician do a complete physical checkup at frequent intervals.
- Drink plenty of fluids, but avoid carbonated drinks or other artificial beverages.
- If you have suffered from kidney stones before, you have to take urine tests on monthly basis that will help to diagnose and check kidney stone formation.
- Never experiment with any kind of medication. Always follow the prescribed medical regime and consult your physician before you make alterations in your dosages.

KIDNEY STONES IN CHILDREN

Kidney stone is a disorder that can affect both adults as well as children. Some kids have a high tendency to develop kidney stones between the ages of 8 to 10 years if this condition is prevalent in their family members. Some external factors also play a crucial role in kidney stone formation in children.

The two major causes of kidney stone occurrences in children are as follows;

Kids tend to drink less water if not persuaded to do so at regular intervals. Due to this the particulate matter in their urine does not get dissolved. Some of these substances found in urine can lead to kidney stone formation.

The general misconception is to provide children with plenty of vitamin supplements in order to facilitate their growth. However, excess consumption of such over-the-counter vitamin and mineral supplements can subsequently lead to kidney stone formation in children.

Urinary tract infection in children is not so rare, yet, it may sometimes lead to kidney stone formation. Infection caused by certain types of bacteria can lead to formation of toxic or residual particulate matter that can eventually lead to kidney stones in children.

Symptoms of kidney stone in children

You have to keep a close watch on your kids and take notice of the ongoing symptoms of kidney stone formation in them. Ask your child whether he or she experiences any abnormal pain or discomfort during urination.

The most common indications of kidney stones in children are as follows;

1. Traces of blood in urine.
2. Severe pain in the lower abdomen or groin during urination.
3. Swelling or pain in the kidney region.
4. Presence of fine sand-like or crystalline matter in urine.

If any of these symptoms persist in your child, then you should seek the help of a specialist immediately. Your doctor will diagnose the child to verify the type of stone and also its severity. He may also verify the family history, medical condition of the child along with his/her eating habits.

A urine test follows right after a thorough physical checkup. Generally, urine sample that has to be examined is nearly twenty-four hours old. Urine test will help the doctor confirm his diagnosis whether the kidney stones in your child's body have been formed as a result of some infection or by external factors.

CT Scans and X-Rays are also used to monitor the course and growth of kidney stones in children. These diagnostic techniques will also reveal any other abnormalities or problems in the child's body that may lead to or contribute to kidney stone formation.

Treatment for kidney stones in children

The most conventional approach to treat kidney stones is to drink plenty of water. This will help remove toxins as well as facilitate the removal of extremely minute kidney stones by dissolving them. If the tests or scans reveal any peculiar type of kidney stone, then the doctor may recommend some diet changes or prescribe some oral medication to help remove such stones. Children love to have junk foods that contain high amounts of sodium. Kids who are prone to kidney stones should be kept away from foods containing high amounts of sodium, artificial flavorings, and oxalates.

If your child is suffering from a very mild case of kidney stone then your physician can refer you to a pediatric urologist who can help remove such stones by medication.

Normally, Lithotripsy method is used to remove stones. In Lithotripsy, sound waves are used to disintegrate the kidney stones into microscopic matter by focusing them onto the child's urinary tract and organ. The kidney stones get removed through urine after undergoing Lithotripsy. It's an extremely painless procedure, however, the child will be given local anesthesia during treatment.

In Ureteroscopy, a small telescope is used instead of sound waves to break down the stone in to smaller fragments. Laparoscopic surgery is also an option for quick removal of kidney stones in children. This procedure involves making three minute incisions in the back through which the kidney stones are removed. After all surgical procedures, a child is kept under medical supervision for at least 24 hours.

When should you start the treatment?

If your child complains about severe pain in back, lower abdomen, groin or exhibits symptoms of discomfort, nausea or persistent fever, you have to consult your physician as soon as possible. Treatment has to be started immediately to relive your child of all such symptoms caused by kidney stone formation. If your child has trouble while passing urine, then it may a clear case of kidney stones. You should also check for traces of pus or blood in the child's urine and give a clear account of your observation to your physician to aid fast diagnosis of kidney stones.

If the tests confirm the stone in child's urinary organ then you should start the prescribed medication or treatment immediately. Normally drugs are sufficient to remove stone from a child's kidney. Children with kidney stone problems may also face like urinary disorders, metabolic disorders, and genetic abnormalities like cystic fibrosis.

The first pediatric center for treatment kidney stones in children is the Children's Hospital of Philadelphia Kidney Stone Center. It is a multifaceted medical facility that helps in prevention and treatment of kidney stones in children. Nowadays, you will come across several such medical institutions all across the globe, that have an efficient team of pediatric urologists to help your child recover from kidney stones.

Kidney stones in children can be a very painful condition; however, it can be easily treated by medication if detected in initial stages. You need not worry about the child's development and overall health after he or she has been treated for kidney stones. Your child will be easily able to continue all of his/her daily activities in a short time right after the kidney stones have been removed.

HOW CHANGES IN DIET CAN HELP, YOU TREAT KIDNEY STONES.

You may wonder how changes in diet can reduce the kidney stone problem. However, most experts believe that wrong food habits and hectic life styles are the main reasons for kidney stone formations. If you are experiencing any peculiar symptoms regarding kidney stones, first seek the help of your doctor to diagnose whether you have kidney stones or not.

If the test confirms kidney stones, then the doctor will prescribe you medication, surgical treatments or even diet plants to help you deal with kidney stones. A registered dietician can help you enjoy a healthy and nutritious diet that can aid you in removal of kidney stones.

What are the diet changes required to pass calcium stones?

The main type of kidney stone that is frequently found in people is the calcium stone. The excessive amounts of calcium deposits do not easily dissolve in urine and can latter result into crystalline residual matter. These crystalline deposits found on the inner walls of the kidney give rise to calcium kidney stones.

Life style changes

The conventional treatment for removing calcium stones involves getting your urine diluted. For this purpose, your body has to be hydrated to adequate levels. Drink plenty of natural fluids or at least twelve glasses of water everyday. You can even include fresh fruit juices in your diet, but try not to take too much of grapefruit juice. If you have a history of kidney stones, then you should avoid foods that contain high amounts of oxalates.

In fact, increase in oxalate levels will facilitate excess calcium absorption in your body that will eventually lead to kidney stone formation. Oxalate is found in certain fruits and vegetables. They are as follows:

- Spinach
- Strawberries- Strawberries are rich in oxalate and hence if you are prone to Kidney Stones you should avoid them.
- Chocolate and other Cocoa products
- Wheat bran
- Nuts
- Beet roots

Restricting or avoiding the above foods will help you to reduce the level of oxalate in your body and help you prevent kidney stones.

A high protein diet is bound to increase the calcium levels in the body. You should consume meat, fish and poultry products in adequate proportions. Similarly, high amounts of sodium increases the calcium excretion process in the body. You have to control the sodium levels in the body in order to prevent kidney stones.

Foods that are high in salt content are as follows:

- Processed meats
- Chips and other snack varieties
- Pickles
- Sauces and gravies
- Tinned soups

These products should be consumed in limited portions in order to avoid formation of calcium stones in the kidneys. Normally, processed and tinned foods contain lot of salt so that the product can have a longer shelf life. Nevertheless, they are harmful to us if consumed too often.

Dairy products like milk, cheese, butter should also be consumed in limited amounts.

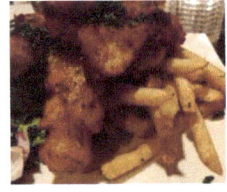 You should also stop taking any unnecessary calcium supplements to check the calcium content entering your body. Apart from this, the doctor may prescribe you medication to help you provide you relief from kidney stone symptoms. Some of these drugs require certain changes in your food habits in order for them to facilitate kidney stone removal.

There are some foods that will cause allergies if taken with the prescribed medication. Hence, you should consult your doctor before taking any kidney stone medication and discuss the required diet plan with him.

Diet changes to pass uric acid stones

Purines have been known to cause Uric acid stones. Alcoholic drinks, dried beans, and peas contain high levels of purines. If you have a habit of prolonged fasting or even if you follow a special diet plant that requires you to stay away from food for long periods of time, then the level of acidity in your body increases. This in turn will cause uric acid stone formation. Uric acid stones can be removed by taking adequate amounts of fresh fruit juices.

Water melon and pomegranate juice are said to be effective in passing the uric acid stones. It is discovered that 8% of people who suffer from kidney stones usually have uric acid stones. It is not an impossible task to remove this stone.

Citrus fruits, apples, tomatoes, strawberries should be avoided to prevent the reoccurrence of uric acid stones. If the above diet changes do not help, the doctor can prescribe you some medication that can relieve you from kidney stone symptoms.

A sedentary life style should be avoided at all costs. Regular exercise such as brisk walking, jogging will definitely help you prevent kidney stone formation in your body.

INTERNATIONAL KIDNEY STONE INSTITUTE

International kidney stone institute is a charitable institution that aims at supporting researches that are focused towards developing the cures and prevent measures for kidney stones. This institution has created a lot of awareness about kidney stones. This organization is also affiliated with the Methodist Hospital and Indiana University of medicine and has earned the reputation of being the best medical facility for dealing with kidney stone diseases.

The IKSI has nearly forty internationally acclaimed scientists who work towards the ambitious goal of eradicating kidney stone diseases.

The objectives supported by the International Kidney Stone Institute are as follows:

Shock wave Lithotripsy Improvement

Shock wave lithotripsy is a common treatment used to remove kidney stones. The scientists in IKSI continue with their research on this subject to improve the safety and success rate of the shock wave treatment. They are also working hard to understand the interconnection between kidney stones and the biological tissues. We can believe that in the near future, the researchers of IKSI will surely improve the effectiveness of the shock wave treatment.

Percutaneous kidney stone removal

Percutaneous lithotripsy treatment is a method of removing kidney stones by making a tiny incision in the back of the patient. The researchers in IKSI are trying to enhance the effectiveness of this treatment and to reduce the risk involved in it. They are doing research in order to improve the techniques used in this treatment so that the quality and success rate will increase.

Randall's Plaque and prevention of stone diseases

Randall's plaque is a mineral deposit formed in the body of patients suffering from calcium oxalate stones. The scientists are performing various researches to diagnose this problem in the patient's body in the early stages and thereby control the kidney stone formation when it is most treatable.

Dietary studies

IKSI is doing various researches to develop specialized diet plans for people who are suffering from kidney stones. In fact, we all know that our diet has large influence on the formation of kidney stones in our bodies. High protein and excessive calcium gets deposited as crystals that develop into kidney stones. These researches will help in getting the required dietary guidance and create awareness among people about the impact of diet in the kidney stone formation. The IKSI scientists are performing researches to provide efficient diet charts, which will help slow down or prevent kidney stone formation.

Kidney stones in the Bariatric population

The researchers in IKSI have found out that the weight loss surgery can adversely affect the PH levels and metabolic equilibrium of the body. Therefore, the chance of getting kidney stone for those who had undergone bariatric surgery is quite high. Scientists are working hard to identify the effects of bariatric surgery on kidney stone formations. This will help people to get some basic information that will help them understand the risks involved in such surgical procedures along with its after effects.

Stone treatment and Hypertension \ Bone disease

Kidney stone disorder will not only affect the functioning of kidneys but also disturb the functioning of some other organs of the urinary tract. There have been certain cases were in the treatment given for kidney stone removal having caused other disorders in patients like Hypertension and Bone diseases. IKSI scientists are doing researches to analyze the risk factors involved in Kidney stone treatment.

What are the preventive steps for Kidney Stones prescribed by IKSI?

In fact, the possibility of kidney stone formation or its reoccurrence cannot be completely avoided, especially when such conditions are the result of inherited or genetic disorders. However, different types of medications as well as surgical procedures can control the frequency and severity of kidney stones. IKSI suggests some the preventive measures to control the kidney stone development.

Every patient suffers from a unique type of Kidney Stone problem. Therefore, to prevent the occurrence of such kidney stones altogether the following points must be considered.

Family history

If there is a family history of kidney stones, the chance of kidney stone formation in any individual increases. Generally, kidney stones such as cystine stones are mainly inherited from the parents or grandparents. You cannot change the genetic problems by taking medication or by resorting to surgical techniques.

However, some prevention methods will help in reduction of the severity of the such diseases. Researches are being conducted to find out the genetic repercussions that can lead to formation of kidney stones in people.

Patient anatomy

Patient anatomy should be considered before prescribing him or her specific preventive measures. Some people become victim of Kidney stones since their kidneys lack the
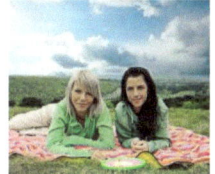 ability of filtering and processing the urine completely. This will induce the deposition of minerals as well as other toxic substances in the kidney. This can result into kidney stones. Therefore, a patient should be examined thoroughly in order to understand the problems.

Stone types

Diagnosing the type of kidney stone will help the doctor suggest effective preventive measures to the patient. The patient can be affected with a single type of kidney stone or a combination of different types of stones. Sometimes a patient may suffer from multiple type kidney stones in different periods of his lifetime. Hence, understanding and diagnosing the type of kidney stone formed is important.

Urine and blood test

Urine and blood test will help us get a better understanding of the type and severity of the prevalent kidney stone. The doctor can get to know about the abnormalities in the patient's body that cause stones. Then some medications can also be prescribed to serve as appropriate preventive methods that will help reduce the kidney stone growth.

Diet history

In most of the cases, the diet intake is responsible for kidney stone formation. Patients can reduce the stone formation by changing the diet and life style. The doctor or a registered dietician will help the patient to change the diet by suggesting what to eat and how much to drink.

Urinary infection history

Urinary tract infections can cause kidney stone formation particularly Stuvite stone formation. If the urine and blood test indicates that the stone formation is a result of urinary tract infection, then special antibiotics will be prescribed to the patient that will eliminate the bacteria that is causing urine infections. Your physician will also suggest some preventive methods in order to avoid consequent infections. If all the suggestions given by the physician are followed, then kidney stone formation will definitely be checked.

Some treatments suggested by IKSI

Researchers at the International Kidney Stone Institution suggest some treatments, which are quite helpful in removing kidney stones. They are as follows:

IKSI specifies that small stones need not require any surgical treatments. Adequate intake of fluids can help pass the small kidney stones out of the body through urine. However, if the stone blocks the urinary tract and causes pain while passing urine, then the patient may require some specific treatment. Pain medication is sometimes more than enough for certain patients. The diet changes and fluid intake will pass the stones.

Surgery is required only if the patient has one kidney or the stone damages the overall functioning of the kidney. It could also be required if the urine flow is totally blocked by the stone. If the stone does not pass within 4 to 6 weeks of medication, then surgery is an inevitable option. IKSI agrees that most of the surgical treatments available to kidney stone affected patients such as Lithotripsy, Ureteroscopy, and Percutaneous stone removal are quite effective.

KIDNEY STONE RESEARCH

Researches in Mayo clinic

Thirty years ago, open surgery was the only surgical treatment to remove kidney stones. The doctor then used to make incisions in the back of the patient and remove the large kidney stone that could not be passed through the urine. This surgery is very risky and had to be performed with utmost caution.

In the year 1981 Mayo clinic first introduced the method of removing kidney stones through percutaneous ultrasonic. In this method, only a tiny incision is made in the back of the patient and a small instrument is inserted into his body to remove the stone.

This method reduces the risk and pain of the open surgery. Again, the patient need only 24 hours of hospitalization. Then he can resume his normal life. Mayo clinic specialists have performed thousands of stone removal procedures each year.

The experienced and qualified Urologists in mayo clinic are doing researches on a regular basis to increase the success rates and to form new technologies to treat kidney stones. Mayo clinic is the number 1 organization in clinical researches on Kidney stone diagnosis, prevention and treatment.

Kidney stone researches at Mayo clinic in Rochester, Minnesota show that there is a close link between diabetes and Kidney stone. People suffering from diabetes have higher chances of getting Uric acid stones and calcium stones that a normal individual. Similarly, people suffering from kidney stones have a risk of developing diabetes. It has been proved that nearly 40% of people with uric acid stones and 9 % of people with calcium stones have diabetes

It is also found that people with kidney stones are more likely to develop Type 2 diabetes than people who do not have any kidney stones.

Some key research findings:

- People who had diabetes for more than 10 years may get Kidney stones.
- People having high blood glucose level frequently have the risk of developing kidney stones.
- People with high blood pressure and high blood fats have the chance of kidney stone growth.
- Smoking tends to increase the risk of kidney stone formation.
- People who have a family history of high blood pressure or kidney diseases have a chance of getting kidney stones.
- Indigenous Australians have a higher tendency to develop kidney stones than others do.

Kidney stone research at Medical College of Wisconsin:

The Kidney stone research group at Medical college of Wisconsin consists of 5 full time faculties, 2 scientists and three PhD Scholars.

Their research activities can be classified into five main categories

1. The research includes the study of epidemiological patterns of the kidney stone disorder. The study also • aims at understanding the impact of age, sex, and ethnicity of a person suffering from kidney stone. The research group also focuses on the reasons for stone recurrence, the disorders caused by medication and surgical treatment to kidney stone and so on.
2. The research group also focuses on the role of injury and it impact on crystal retention.
3. The research scholars have found out that calcium oxalate stones have close relation to hypertension.
4. They also found that recurrent calcium stone formation is mainly due to genetic reasons.
5. The research also focuses on the oral oxalate ingestion and its link to calcium oxalate crystalluria. The study also shows that the stone recurrence is associated with age, sex, ethnicity and geographical location of the patient.

The division of Kidney diseases Of National Institute of diabetes, Digestive and kidney diseases (NIDDK) focuses on researches for treatment and prevention for kidney stones. New medication and lithotripsy treatments have made kidney stone removal easier. However, NIDDK researches are doing some researches to get answer to the following questions:

- Why some people suffer from more pain due to kidney stones while others do not?
- How can a doctor predict that his patients have are prone to kidney stones?
- Are there any side effects of lithotripsy? If so, how long the side effects will last?
- What is the role of genes in kidney stone formation?
- What is the substance found in urine that can prevent the formation of kidney stones?

The researchers of NIDDK are also trying to develop new medicines for the treatment of kidney stones that has fewer side effects.

HOW TO MANAGE KIDNEY STONE DISEASE?

Follow-up consultation is necessary to prevent kidney stone formation. This is particularly important for young adults and children. If you have suffered from the pain of kidney stones earlier in your lifetime, then stand at a higher risk of developing them again. Therefore, follow up and a routine test along with some specialized tests becomes essential. Tests include blood and urine tests along with X-rays and CT scans. This will help the doctor to analyze the risk factors, which tend to promote recurrent stone formation.

Management of kidney stones involves two aspects- diet and medication. The doctor can advise you about the diet and medication regimes after analyzing the type of kidney stone you suffer from.

Some of kidney stone management techniques are as follows:

Lifestyle changes

If you have been diagnosed with kidney stones, then you should start drinking more water or fluids. Drinking 10 to 12 glasses of water is recommended in order to check kidney stone formation. However, you not include coffee, tea and colas or other artificial beverages in your diet. You should minimize salt consumption as sodium is one of the major cause of kidney stones.

The average salt intake per day should not exceed 2000 to 3000 milligram. That means you should not take more than one-tablespoon salt daily.

Taking minimum amount of calcium and animal proteins will be more beneficial. Six ounces of fish, meats or poultry products are enough to sustain an average human being. These 6 ounces must be consumed separately by dividing them into two meals daily.

White flour products like Pizza will increase the risk of stone formation. Hence you should limit the consumption of such items.

Rich oxalate food like Instant coffee, beets, spinach and other dark green leaf vegetables should be consumed in limited quantity .The total vitamins required per day are 100%. Do not consume more than the prescribed dosages.

Medications

If you develop kidney stones after making dietary changes, then your doctor can prescribe some medication to remove these kidney stones.

Medication is however, required to help dissolve these kidney stones and to control pain. The following medication will help you in passing small stones by dissolving them;

Hydrochlorothiazide

This drug is normally used to remove calcium oxalate and phosphate stones. It helps to decrease the calcium absorption in the urine. The medicine is effective when the person takes a low sodium diet.

Potassium citrate

This will help in boosting citrate content in the urine. This in turn will help in reducing the growth of calcium oxalate stones.

Allopurinol

This medicine is prescribed to reduce uric acid in the body and thereby to control the uric acid stone formation in kidney.

Prophylactic antibiotics

This drug will help in preventing Urinary tract infections. It is already known that stuvite stone is only formed due to urinary tract infection.

Pencillamine, thiola and Cuprimine

These drugs will control the growth of Cystine stones. These medications may produce some side effects. Therefore, the doctor should clearly monitor the health status of the patient on a regular basis.

Hyperparathyroidism Treatment

The parathyroid glands are overactive for people suffering from Hyperparathyroidism and this condition can lead to kidney stone formation. The parathyroid glands will be located in four corners of the thyroid gland.

One of the gland produces too much of calcium. As a result, the calcium will be deposited as crystals and then develop into kidney stones.

Surgical treatment for Hyperparathyroidism will also be essential to cure kidney stone disorder. However, the surgery must be performed by an endocrine surgeon and not by an Urologist.

TIPS TO AVOID KIDNEY STONES

Kidney stone sometimes cause acute pain. The pain seems to increase in summer or in dry climate. Extreme sweating, spicy and fried foods will aggravate the symptoms caused by kidney stones.

- You can avoid spicy foods to control kidney stone problem.
- People who live in hot weather conditions tend to develop kidney stones during summer. Kidney stone specialists have suggested some tips to prevent kidney stone formation in such conditions.
- We all know taking water in adequate quantities is the best way to avoid kidney stones. However, do not take mineral water. Drink plain water.
- You can take lemonades and natural concoctions.
- Most of the physicians specify that grape fruit juice can increase the risk of kidney stone formation. Hence, avoid grape fruit juice if you are suffering from kidney stones.
- Always try to stay healthy and hydrated.
- Restrict the use of sodium.
- Meat and artificial sauces should be reduced in diet.

Summer is the crucial period which tends to be a main factor which can only help in the formation of kidney stones. Take more fluids in summer including fresh fruit juices to prevent stone formation.

Men are more likely to suffer from kidney stones than women, the reason is quite simple. Men generally end up staying all the day in heat and then after they go home they take spicy and oily foods in their meals, thus increasing the risk of kidney stone formation. Therefore, avoid fried foods and junk foods, at least in summer. Try to maintain your blood pressure at normal levels. This will help in reducing the risk of kidney stone development.

Dehydration is common in summer particularly among children. You should be careful to avoid such episodes that in turn will help to prevent kidney stone formation. Take lot of fiber-rich foods like oats, beans, cereals, carrots etc. Eat beef and pork in limited quantity.

Eating high amounts of red meat has been known to increase the risk of kidney stone formations. Therefore, try to avoid red meat as much as possible.

WHAT ARE THE SIDE EFFECTS INVOLVED IN THE MEDICATION FOR KIDNEY STONES?

Potassium citrate

Potassium citrate is administered in proportionate dosages to control calcium stones. The results indicate that it is nearly 95% successful in removing calcium kidney stones. There are possibilities of occurrence of few side effects like vomiting, gas and diarrhea.

Orthophosphate

Orthophosphate is almost similar to Potassium citrate. It helps check the growth of calcium stones in kidneys. The possible side effects are gas and diarrhea.

Thiazides

This medication is effective in controlling calcium stone growth particularly when dietary changes are not at all helpful.

However, it has some side effects:

- Potassium level may be decreased in blood.
- Frequent urination.
- Erection problem in men.
- If the patient has Gout problems, then the symptoms may worsen.
- Similarly, if the patient has diabetes, the symptoms may also worsen.

Tiopronin

This may help in preventing cystine stones. However, it causes many side effects that include:

- Yellowish color skin
- Rashes in skin
- Kidney damage.
- Blood cells production may be decreased in bone marrow.
- Joint pain.

Over Dosage of medication will cause number of problems,. Hence always avoid taking medicine without medical supervision in case of treatments of kidney stones. Since the medication for stones are known to have peculiar side effects, over dosage may lead to severe problems and even kidney failure.

Urease inhibitors

This will help in preventing stuvite stones. The possible side effects are as follows:

- Head ache
- Constipation or diarrhea
- Vomiting
- Depression
- Rashes in skin
- Excessive sweating
- Anemia
- Pulmonary embolism.

Yet there are only a few side effects caused by the Urease Inhibitors, they have been proven to be beneficial for the process of removing kidney stones. But before you opt for them, you should consult your doctor before taking any medication. The doctor can prescribe you other drugs or give you tips in order to help you to reduce the side effects of this medication.

Some drugs will be effective only if you follow a particular diet plan. Your doctor or a registered dietician can help you design an effective nutritional plan for this purpose.

HOMEOPATHIC APPROACH TO REMOVE KIDNEY STONES

The number of kidney stone sufferers has been steadily increasing on a daily scale. Medication is effective to treat such kidney stones but it may cause side effects as mentioned above. Homeopathy is an alternative therapy that provides a natural way to pass kidney stones. However, if the stone is too large or too complicated to remove, then surgery will be the only possible method to remove such kidney stones.

Some Homeopathy remedies

Like any approach, Homeopathy also suggests increasing the daily fluid intake in order to prevent kidney stone formation. Drinking more water will help to pass the stones on their own. You can even pass urine forcibly and speedily so that the stone will come down fast. Suppose if you experience severe pain, Homeopathy has plenty of pain management drugs. Such drugs include Beri beri vulgaris, Lycopodium, Uva ursi and so on.

Homeopathy not only cures pain but also removes stones permanently. As there are no side effects involved, people are switching over to this approach nowadays. This approach uses the body's own healing power to deal problems caused by kidney stone formation. Hence, you will be relieved of all your kidney stone problems without having to undergo surgical procedures or experience any side effects. Since injections and surgery are not used in this method, you will get a really safe and effective cure for your kidney stones.

Another important benefit in Homeopathy is that it reduces the tendency to form kidney stones. Most of the approaches used to treat kidney stones will not aid in prevention of the recurrence of stones. But, Homeopathy will help you to get permanent and long term relief. Most of the Homeopathy remedies are available in pellet form with lactose base. If you have an allergy to milk and milk products, Homeopathic tinctures or liquids can also be used.

HERBAL REMEDY FOR KIDNEY STONES

Apart from the above approaches, herbal remedies are also available in for treating kidney stones. Kidney Dr. is one of the herbal products available in the market which will prevent kidney stone formation. It is 100% natural.

The product contains the mixture of herbs used in various countries to aid all types of kidney problems. This can be used in diluted form and taken with water or juice. You can even give it to children, but make sure they are not allergic to such substances.

Within 3 to 6 weeks you are bound to experience a difference in your overall health by making use of herbal remedies. Small stones will be passed through urine within 3 weeks by such natural remedies.

Herbs can help in passing small stones easily and without any side effects.

Naturopathy is helpful in removal of small kidney stones. There is no pain or side effects involved in this treatment. It is safe as well as effective. Nowadays, herbs are available in perfect mixtures that have been crafted into easy- to-take capsule form.

This will help you to remove stones without pain and side effects. In fact, Herbal remedies also include effective analgesics and antipyretics. This will also improve the overall health of the patient.

Naturopathy treatment includes nutritional recommendation along with herbs. Some food may cause allergies if taken along with these herbs. Hence, you should seek the help of a Naturopathy specialist to know about the correct diet plan to be followed while undergoing naturopathic treatment for kidney stones. In fact, a proper diet will support kidney functioning and discourage stone formation. Natural therapies are available to ease the pain while treating kidney stones.

Some herbal medicines that cure kidney stones are as follows:

1. Cleavers - This is a very powerful herb can effectively cure kidney stones.
2. Kava kava - This has the capacity of providing slight sedation and thus, provides relief from pain. Therefore, by using kava kava a person can get relief from certain symptoms of kidney stones. This herb is used with a combination of other herbs as well.
3. Seven barks - This is an effective sedative and can help a kidney stone patient calm down and relax. It helps in checking kidney stone problems.
4. Gravel root - This is very effective herb which helps in the removal of small kidney stones as well as the gravel formed in the kidney.

Along with the herbal remedies, a proper and balanced diet should be taken. Naturopathy prescribes a high fiber diet to pass kidney stones easily.

It is also advised to take water to the minimum of 50 % of the total body weight. You should also avoid sugar, alcohol, beverages, refine white flour products etc. Brown rice, banana, oats as well some other grains.

These approaches are effective in removing small stones only. Large and complicated stones must be removed by way of surgery. Kidney stone is a curable condition if discovered in initial stages. Make some small changes in your life style and diet and lead a healthy life free of kidney stones.

KIDNEY STONE FOUNDATION

Kidney stone foundation, Canada

Kidney stone foundation Canada states that one out of ten Canadians has the risk of kidney stone formation. It is increasing day by day irrespective of age, gender and geographical location. However, people living in hot climate are more prone to kidney stone formation. This is because these people tend to lose more water through sweating and therefore they need to drink more fluid especially water.

Kidney stone foundation, Canada focuses on people suffering from kidney stones and the researches prove that people with high blood pressure have more chances of getting kidney stones.

Kidney stone foundation Canada specifies some common causes for stone formation

- People who are taking less amounts of fluids, have a higher risk of getting stones.
- People who are taking plenty of vitamin and mineral supplements along with a lot of dairy products are at a greater risk of developing kidney stones.
- People who are living in hot weather conditions and drink very little water are bound to develop kidney stones.
- People who take large doses of vitamin c are also prone to kidney stone formation.
- People who take high oxalate foods more face the risk of stone formation.
- Kidney foundation Canada specifies the following symptoms as kidney stone symptoms.
- Severe pain in the back and abdomen for a long period of time.
- Nausea and vomiting.
- Blood and pus in urine.

Kidney stone foundation in Canada specifies that the size of the kidney stone normally varies from a sand grain to a golf ball. The bigger the size of the kidney stone, the more complicated is the process of treatment.

National Kidney foundation

National Kidney foundation funds many researches to focus on kidney stone problems and their treatments. The researchers of NKF focus mainly on kidney stone problems.

Diet suggested by national kidney stone foundation is as follows;

The NKF suggests taking lot of water everyday. Every doctor will advise you to take lot of fluids but how much is always a question. National kidney foundation specifies that taking two glasses of water in excess every day is required to prevent and pass kidney stones.

Treatment suggested by National Kidney Foundation

National kidney foundation agrees that Lithotripsy is the best method of removing kidney stones. Here sound waves are focused in the back of the patient's body so that the location of the stone is confirmed. This process can identify even small stones. Then the stone is removed by treating it with pulses of sound waves. The patient is given local or general anesthesia while undergoing this treatment.

Advantages of Lithotripsy

This method has the main advantage of removing stones within 30 minutes. The patient requires hospitalization for only one day. He can resume his normal activities within a short period of time. The small stone in urinary tract can be easily removed in this method.

Disadvantages of Lithotripsy

This method is a bit expensive, yet this method fails to remove complicated stones. The surgeon needs to use another method along with lithotripsy to get rid of kidney stones altogether. Therefore, this procedure is regarded to be somewhat complicated.

Since this method does not remove small stone pieces, it causes discomfort for the patient while passing them through urine. This is the main disadvantage of this method.

LASER SURGERY FOR REMOVING KIDNEY STONES

In laser surgery method, the surgeon will insert a microscopic telescope into the patients' body to locate the stone. Then he will use a laser beam of fixed intensity to disintegrate the kidney stones. The stone will then be removed with the help of a basket that is attached to this telescope. This method is simple and requires anesthesia. The patient will experience immediate relief after this surgery and can resume his daily activities in a few hours.

Advantages of Laser surgery

Laser surgery never causes any pain or discomfort to the patient. Therefore, lots of kidney stone sufferers are switching to laser surgery. Again, the patient does not require any hospitalization.

The patient can resume his or her normal life immediately after this procedure. If you don't have much time to spare from your busy and hectic schedules, then this procedure is ideal for you.

Disadvantages of laser surgery

The laser surgery is costlier than any other treatment and hence it is not affordable by all. This is the main disadvantage of this procedure.

Again if the stones are more complicated to remove with laser surgery, the patient can then go for Percutaneous treatment.

Endoscope laser surgery is also suggested for treating kidney stones. This is also a costly method of removing kidney stones.

EASY STEPS TO PREVENT THE RISK OF KIDNEY STONE FORMATION

Though there are number of treatments available to cure kidney stone, it is always better to prevent it. Some easy steps to prevent kidney stones are as follows:

Step 1: As already stated, drink plenty of water. This will help you to stay hydrated. Water is the best and cheapest form of treatment to cure kidney stones. Drink lot of fresh fruit juices along with water.

Step 2: Eat lots of fiber rich foods such as Wheat bran, oats, carrots and cabbage are rich in fiber and you can take it to avoid constipation. This in turn will help you to prevent kidney stones.

Step 3: Avoid high oxalate containing foods like tea, instant coffee, carbonated drinks, colas etc. These things can lead to kidney stone formation.

Step 4: You should avoid calcium rich foods. Dairy products should be consumed in limited quantity only.

Step 5: You should take limited quantities of sodium. Sodium will cause dehydration and thereby promote kidney stone formation.

Step 6: Always avoid fried food. This will increase the acidity in the urine. If you do eat fried food, consume it in limited quantities.

If you manage your groceries, it can help you prevent kidney stones. You just have to spend a little more on your grocery bill. Always buy some beverages and vegetable puree from local grocery shop that have no preservatives in them. This will help these juices can help break down kidney stones that will be eventually passed through the urine.

Pepper, Cumin seeds etc are good for digestion. You can add it with onion or cucumber. This will help to prevent constipation. This in turn will reduce the risk of kidney stone formation.

Dehydration and Kidney stones

Dehydration to high extents can definitely lead to kidney stones. People get dehydrated when they lose fluid from their body and are not able to replenish its quantities. Diarrhea and vomiting may cause dehydration in children. This will definitely lead to kidney stone formation.

Babies and the elderly folk are more prone to dehydration. If you take your children to places which are hot or arid, then make sure that they are given plenty of fluids.

KIDNEY STONE ANALYSIS

Kidney stone analysis is required when:

- The person experiences severe pain in the back or abdomen.
- If traces of blood or pus is found in the urine.
- If the urine has a distinctly foul smell.
- The person has frequent urinary tract infections.
- The person has abnormally shaped kidneys.

Kidney stone analysis will help the doctor to understand the type of stone and to start the treatment.

The kidney stone analysis also helps the doctor to develop the specific diet plan and medication regimes. These tests include x-ray tests, urine test and blood tests.

Urine sample is generally preferred to test for kidney stones. This would help in analyzing the type of stone and also decide appropriate treatments that can be used to remove such kidney stones. If the stone is complicated and large, the doctors will advice you to go to an Urologist.

HOME TREATMENT FOR REMOVING KIDNEY STONE

Often home treatments and remedies are enough to treat small and uncomplicated kidney stones. A balanced diet along with the adequate amounts of fluids will help you to pass the kidney stones easily. However, if you experience pain due to kidney stones continuously then are bound to feel frustrated. You can take pain medication to relieve such symptoms.

You can take some self medication to control pain. Non-steroidal medicines like aspirin and ibuprofen is sometimes enough to manage the pain caused by kidney stones. If you feel extreme pain while passing urine, then the doctor will advice you to take some strong pain control pills.

The doctors will advice you to use a strainer while passing urine. This will help to filter sand or gravel in urine. The doctor will analyze the stone to know the type of stone. He will also suggest some diet change according to the type of stone.

You may feel more pain when the stone moves in the urinary tract system. After this stage home treatment will give the desired results and in such cases, stronger medications or surgery is recommended.

Your doctor may suggest some treatment like lithotripsy or shock wave treatment depending on the condition of the stone.

In rare cases open surgery is advised. However, open surgery has been rarely used since the introduction of laser surgery and lithotripsy.

CONCLUSION

We have discussed about the causes, treatments and diet changes required for removing kidney stones. Kidney stone is not a dreadful disease. It is manageable with medication. However, the pain is more in this disease. Many women complain that such pain is similar to pain experienced during childbirth. Therefore, it is better to take steps for prevention rather than to rush in for medications and surgery.

One must consume atleast 8-10 glasses of water. Avoid fried and junk foods. Eat healthy and live healthy. Some regular exercises on a daily basis will keep you mentally and physically fit. Sedentary life style will increase the risk of stone formation. Prevention is any day better than cure.

www.ingramcontent.com/pod-product-compliance
Lightning Source LLC
Chambersburg PA
CBHW041507280526
45792CB00004B/1169